Goodbye to Pain

Antony Sherry

Table of Contents

Prologue

This book is my story, and I hope that you, the reader, will understand more about pain and my way of addressing this often-tricky issue. It contains information on how I treated my chronic pain, which could be an option for you.

This book will inform you about some of the things I have learned along the way. I'm passionate about helping people and animals to become pain-free or at least diminish the pain to a manageable level to improve their quality of life.

If you know me, you'll know I love a good cup of coffee. A lot of coffee went into making this book and chatting about it. Make yourself a nice drink, sit back, and enjoy.

About the Author

Tony Sherry is an experienced nurse and complementary therapist treating both people and animals with muscular issues and getting excellent results.

His exploration of complementary therapies started following a horse-riding accident accident in 2011, resulting in severe chronic back pain which conventional treatments could not alleviate. He was surviving on painkillers.

In 2016, he resigned from his job as a matron in the National Health Service to start his business as a complementary therapist, ECH Therapies, hoping to make a difference to the quality of life of people and animals experiencing pain and discomfort.

He tailors his treatment according to each individual's needs, meaning that each treatment is unique and customised. His love for animals is obvious, and the way the animals interact with him is heart-warming to behold.

To enquire about booking Tony for lectures and demonstrations at an event, email him at tony@echtherapies.co.uk.

Acknowledgements

Goodbye to Pain is my first book, and it was something that I had never planned. Writing has not always been easy when doing everything else I have to do in my business.

I am grateful to Dom Hodgson my business coach for encouraging me to write the book.

I'm thankful for each client that I have the privilege of helping, as I learn so much with each session. Some have contributed beautiful testimonials to include in the book.

I want to thank my life partner, John Rea, for being there when I had doubts that I would finish the book or whether anyone would even read it.

1.

Introduction

There was a time in my life that seemed disastrous. I felt as if I was losing everything because of the pain in my back. The happy times in my life seemed a distant memory, and there were times when I felt as if I was at the end of the road with no future ahead. I was in so much pain with no relief from it day or night despite taking loads of medication and consulting professionals, both of which I thought would help me regain my old self and my wonderful life. If they had told me to "hang from the ceiling wearing an Aqua-Lung" (thanks to Kenneth Williams in *Carry on Nurse* for that beautiful description), I would have, as I thought they had the knowledge and experience to rid me of this debilitating pain. Unfortunately, it was not the case.

In the summer of 2011, I found myself strapped to a spinal board in the back of a slow-moving ambulance, and that day, my life changed.

I was riding my big and relatively young horse around the arena at a horse show. Just as I asked the horse to go into a canter, the unexpected happened. Three children jumped up from behind a hedge screaming, and it frightened my horse so much that he gave me a lesson in rodeo riding! With all the bucking, I flew through the air and landed on the base of my spine.

I remember the panic well: Where was my horse? Was he galloping off into the distance? What the hell had happened?   I tried to get up and felt the most searing pain I had ever experienced. I was in total agony. People rushed over to help me, but I found I could not move. An ambulance arrived, and they gave me gas and moved me onto a spinal board. I felt every bump as we drove across the field and on the road to the hospital. Pain seized my body at each bump, and I didn't know what to do. Was this a serious injury? Would I get over this? After x-rays, I was diagnosed with soft tissue damage in my back, and the doctor discharged me home to rest with regular pain killers. If only that had been the problem and the pain had been resolved!

I'm better now, much to my doctor's surprise....but how?

The relentless pain I found myself in made me take painkillers as if they were smarties. Everything I tried to do caused pain. A good night's sleep was impossible because I had to brace myself and concentrate hard on turning over with the least amount of pain and not waking my partner up. I could not walk without a walking stick. I felt and looked like a 90-year-old man, and I was only 49 at the time. This relentless pain and lack of sleep took a toll on my mental health. Was my life going to be like that from then on? Was that as good as it could get, or would I get worse? Why wouldn't the pain just go away? Would I have to give up work? Why me? At that point, it was definitely the pain that ruled my life and dictated what I could do. Some days, I did not want to move for fear of it getting worse.

Three weeks after the accident, I was not any better, and a general practitioner (GP) I saw at the time said that as I was over 40, I should resign myself to the fact that I would need to learn how to live with the pain for the rest of my life. I was devastated, and all those negative thoughts flooded back into my head (crap, this was it, I had been written off). Deep inside my head, a little voice refused to believe it, and the GP's words were like a red rag to a bull. He organised some physiotherapy sessions for me, but I was only allowed six appointments, and if I needed more, I would need to pay privately, but this would take a few weeks to organise.

The GP finished the consultation, suggesting that I could try acupuncture, as it often works for back pain, and someone in the village practised it. This person had treated the GP, and it seemed to work well for him.

Acupuncture was a lifeline thrown at me. Could this glimmer of hope turn the tide?

I saw the acupuncturist a couple of days later. Paul inserted the needles into me and left the room. The next thing, I knew was being startled as the door opened again. He had been gone for 15 minutes, and I bloody well fell asleep. When I stood up, I thought I was dreaming, as the intensity of the pain had dropped from a 10 to 3. I felt so happy that it had worked, and I felt much more comfortable. I looked in the mirror and noticed I was standing straighter than I had in weeks. I slept so well that night. It was astonishing. However, a few days later, the pain level crept up, so I returned, and once again, the pain dropped to a tolerable level.

My first physiotherapy appointment arrived. I had been looking forward to this so much, as I wanted to be on the road to recovery.

They would rid me of all the pain for good, or so I thought. It took a lot of effort to get there in the first place, as I was in a lot of pain that day, but I forced myself to do so because I wanted to be pain-free. When they called my name, I felt like a kid going to meet Santa, so excited was I. The physio asked my medical history and then looked at my back and said, "Oh, your back's in spasm. I can't do anything to it while it's like that."

I was shocked, stunned, and so disappointed as no help could be offered to me. It felt like a kick in the teeth, as if the medical profession had let me down.

I was advised to go home, to keep gulping painkillers, and to put a hot water bottle on my back until our second appointment the following week.

The following week, I returned to the physio department with my fingers crossed. They examined my back again and declared, "Your back is still in spasm. I can't do anything to it while it's like that. Let's try again next week."

I felt so angry and frustrated because it took so much organising, pain, and effort to get to the hospital to be told they couldn't touch me. It felt as if my life was being flushed down the toilet. Was the amount of pain I was experiencing worth trying to attend another appointment only to be told they couldn't touch me? I decided not, as I thought it was a waste of time for both the physio and myself. I went back for an acupuncture appointment, which again reduced the pain to a tolerable level.

Then I started thinking: if acupuncture eased my pain, what else out there could help me? Was there a treatment out there that could permanently rid me of the pain?

So, I searched the Internet to see what could help me. I felt old and extremely cynical when looking at other therapies because I thought that if something worked on me, then it did work. I was not really into all this hippy tree-hugging stuff.

I researched alternative/complementary therapies. I

spent hours and days sifting through different websites, articles, and YouTube videos on my desktop.

One therapy I came across was the Australian EMMETT Technique. I could find very little on it, but the one thing that stood out was the claim of light finger pressure, even on clothes, producing instant effects and treating anybody anywhere. At that time, my thoughts about it were, "What a load of utter bollocks!" I shut down my computer and did not give it any further thought.

I am pain-free now, but how? I hear you ask. I will explain this later.

I find pain fascinating, as it can have so many components. Moreover, everybody who experiences pain does so differently. People who suffer from the same injury describe the pain in their own way, resulting in many different meanings for the same thing. Perhaps, some or all of my story so far resonates with you to some degree.

2.

Acute and Chronic Pain

This chapter will explain why we experience pain and the differences between acute and chronic pain. Understanding it better will help you grasp the complexity of the subject, but please remember you are not alone in your experience of pain. For this book, I am only using the terms acute and chronic pain. There are many other types of pain, but I want to try and keep things as simple as possible.

Why do we feel pain? Pain is a complex physiological and psychological response to some event. Pain is a significant warning of possible harm, and it makes us move away from the cause.

Pain alters our behaviour by compelling us to withdraw from the painful stimulus, and it's the same for animals. This behavioural change can also act as a social cue to avoid the trigger. Animals in a pack or herd will run from anything that may cause harm.

By acting as a warning signal and alerting us to possible tissue damage, the resulting behaviour of pain avoidance may evoke a wide variety of actions in response.

Physiologically, pain occurs when the sensory nerve endings (pain receptors) contact the stimulus causing the pain, such as a leg when being kicked in the shin or a burn.

In an article published in the British Medical Journal (1) in 2016, which was a meta-analysis of population studies, the author suggested that chronic pain affects between one-third and half of the population of the UK. This mind-blowing figure corresponded to about 28 million adults at the time of writing this book.

A meta-analysis is a quantitative, epidemiological study designed to examine previous research studies that discuss conclusions. A rigorously conducted meta-analysis is a helpful tool in evidence- based medicine and may investigate a particular drug treatment to examine its effectiveness.

The British Pain Society (2) in 2021 estimated that 8 million adults in the UK report having chronic moderate-to-severe disabling pain. They estimated that back pain alone accounts for 40% of sickness in the NHS, and the potential cost to the UK economy is £10 billion.

The website statistic.com (3) estimates that there will be 24 million dogs and cats in the UK in 2021. Moreover, over 7 million animals experience chronic pain in the UK. However, animals can't express pain the same way people can, which complicates things a little. Nonetheless, as a therapist, I can understand what's going on through observation.

Pain is an area of practice that I find fascinating. Helping somebody, be it a person or an animal, trapped in an awful cycle of pain, which, in a majority of cases, adversely affects mental health, is something I find satisfying. I can look into someone's eyes and see and feel the level of darkness looking back at me because I have been there. When I come across this, I have to talk to the client about my own experience with pain. I see their face change as I talk about a pain issue that limits every activity you try to carry out and how it's mentally draining and physically exhausting. Chronic or constant pain will be on a person's mind 24 hours a day, seven days a week. The brain slips into survival mode and tries to compensate for the way it holds the body and the way the muscles move to avoid more pain. For every movement or activity undertaken by the pain sufferer, the brain thinks to itself, "Now how can we do this with the least amount of pain?" Going to the toilet will be difficult and painful, so you don't drink and eat much to avoid the activity. Turning over in bed can be difficult without bracing yourself or holding onto the headboard. Thus, you never get proper sleep and wake up as tired as when you went to bed. I'm sure you can understand how exhausting this can be, and when we are tired, it lowers our pain threshold further. When I talk to the client and explain all of this, I see the look in their eyes that shows they know they are not alone in this and are not the only person suffering in this way. Demonstrating empathy and understanding builds a great bond between the client and myself.

Pain can make us feel so helpless when it's relentless, and no progress is being made to alleviate it. We will need the help of medication and pain killers, but again when this doesn't help, this affects our mental health. So many different types of medication are available today, and it can be easy to become dependent on them. When I was in chronic pain, I used to dread running out of painkillers even though they did not work very well on me. The pain wore me down so much that I would cry at the drop of a hat and sometimes for no apparent reason.

Chronic or long-term pain is experienced differently by those who suffer from it. Backs, necks, and shoulders are the most common things I see and treat. I find this awful type of pain extremely challenging. How do I undo some of the clients' brains' strategies to move and operate with the least amount of discomfort? I have to explain a lot to people, and I may have to gently repeat things more than once to challenge and change their way of thinking, and this demands patience and time. I have to change the client's muscles and then allow the body to adjust. If I rush in and change a lot suddenly, the body and the brain will go into overload.

I feel that mental health is not acknowledged by many pain sufferers for all sorts of different reasons, and it certainly is not because they are weak. However, if you have been told that nothing can be done for your pain and that you need to keep taking the painkillers, it will considerably affect you as a person and can be life-defining.

However, constant consumption of pain killers can be the new norm of life for the client. Things can get back to as near usual as possible, or with some adaptation and determination, things can be a little better but nowhere near before the pain started.

The brain is the most impressive organ and can reset itself to this new normal of compensation within the body very quickly. This process can continue even if the initial injury has completely healed. The brain remembers the awful pain it has experienced and does everything to prevent it from going back there. I like to think of it as a muscle that has a memory – it knows where it should be and how it should move but develops a false memory when the body compensates.

Mindset can be a big issue for some people regarding the pain/ discomfort or a restricting movement problem. We all know that bearing a negative outlook can make things feel worse. We live in a society where negative stories sell newspapers or make us stop and think, so we unconsciously dwell on the negative. When it comes to managing pain, Buddha's well-known words written many centuries ago still ring true today: how you think about your pain can change how you feel it, for better or worse.

The subject of positive thinking in pain management has been widely studied, especially in chronic pain. I find this awful type of pain extremely challenging. Research has proven that negative thinking worsens pain or inhibits a person's ability to cope.

Over the years, I have seen how attitude can affect people so many times, especially in a hospital setting, when someone has been in intensive care for a long time. The patient often feels helpless and trapped, as they have no energy and every movement hurts. They need assistance with everything. Consequently, the nurse should ensure that the patient has enough painkillers and should be the voice of positivity and help them create a new focus. Raising the patient's spirits can and does affect the length of hospital stay.

As you can see from my description above, this can be an intricate web that the brain and muscles weave together. My job is to help the client's brain and muscles unentangle this dependency to the best of my ability and regain what they have lost. Sometimes this does not work out as I would want it to, but that could mean that other factors are involved.

I had a client a few years ago that asked me if I could help her with her neck problem. She had been involved in a road traffic accident 15 years before, following which she had been in pain and had been unable to rotate her head to the left. She had been examined by numerous doctors and had done every scan you can think of and had spent a great deal of money on several types of therapy to try and get rid of the pain and restore movement. I assessed her neck, and when I asked her to turn her head to the left, she couldn't and turned from the hips. She then admitted that she found driving uncomfortable and made her husband drive whenever she could. Her way of thinking about her neck had turned negative, and she had almost given up thinking it could or would change.

I performed two corrections, one on the shoulders and another on the neck. I then asked if she would turn her head to the left, and she did, and her hips stayed still. The look on her face was so funny. With her head touching her left shoulder, she stared at me and declared, "You're a witch." She then asked me to take a photo of her, as her husband of 10 years had never seen her neck in that position. That only took me two minutes, and it's been perfect ever since.

My approach to pain management is that it's a very individual thing, and no two bodies ever experience pain in precisely the same way. With this in mind, I cannot treat everyone the same way (one pill does not fit all). I cannot treat everyone with a shoulder issue with the same care package. Each person is an individual and should be treated with respect to the uniqueness of their body and problem. One of my pet dislikes is when healthcare professionals treat people or animals as if they were on a conveyer belt, and it's the same for everyone with that issue. My time as a nurse taught me that there might be some similarities in the way people experience pain, but we are all different and have different needs to sort the pain out.

With the right approach from the client and therapist, the pain will significantly reduce or be completely eliminated. Reducing the level of pain or making the pain vanish could change someone's life in so many ways and bring the biggest smile you have ever seen to a face. That, to me, is worth all the tea in China and gives me the best feeling ever. Yes, it does take a positive attitude to want to change things for people, but the beauty of treating animals is that they are not like that. If I change the pain or take it away from animals, they become my new best friend within a minute or two. I have often treated horses and dogs that other therapists and vets won't touch. I take my time introducing myself to the animal and letting it understand that I'm not a vet and will not be sticking a needle in them. It's a well-known fact that many animals don't like going to the vet's clinic or seeing a vet in their stable, and if they do, they become stressed and very anxious. When I touch the animal where they need help, and the tension in the muscle slips away, they give me a look, as if asking me, "What have you just done?" I also get the best thank you from them when they will lick my hand or want a cuddle.

Pain in animals is perhaps even more complex than in people. The physical processes of how pain is sensed and experienced are similar in animals and people. It's known that animals feel pain, and we are all aware of this, but we don't understand particularly well how they experience pain, and animals can't verbalise their pain in the same way as people can. Still, domesticated animals rely on people to observe their pain and recognise and evaluate its severity and impact.

Many studies in various domestic animals indicate that animals who have had surgery but have not been provided adequate pain relief demonstrate behaviours that suggest pain is being experienced. When pain medication was administered, these behaviours changed.

I was asked to treat a horse who had known anger issues. The horse had broken two vets' arms when they were asked to see him, as his behaviour had changed and he was now aggressive. When I arrived at the yard, a staff member walked the horse around, and I saw that he was not a happy boy. The head groom told me that all this had occurred within the last four months. Until four months ago, he was a gentle, lovely gelding. She then told me that the horse did not like going into a stable, did not like being tied up, did not like being groomed, and hated men. My life was flashing in front of my eyes, and I thought, "Oh crap, what have I let myself in for."

I gently got hold of the horse's lead rope and touched him on the top of the shoulders. With that, he stood still and looked at me. then I repeated the same thing, and he leaned into my fingers. Within a few minutes, he was like a lamb and licking my neck.

After a few more corrections, he was happy to go into a stable and went home a couple of days later with no issues at all. He had been trying to tell people he was in discomfort/pain, and people were not listening to him, so he thought to himself, "How else can I let them know!"

The words we use matter, and I have learnt this through experience and lessons over the years. The client may have been to multiple therapists before meeting me, which I consider a bonus, as some of my work has already been carried out. It can be devastating news when someone has been told that nothing more can be done for their pain or discomfort. This phrase is lodged in their head, and they go away thinking that the issue becomes a self-fulfilling prophecy. If the healthcare professional said that there was nothing more that they could offer the client, that would not have such a negative impact.

There are ways of having a conversation with a client

and using probing questions to find out where the matter sits in people's heads. Where have they had an unfavourable opinion given to them and by who? I then ask the million-dollar questions "Do you want to feel better?" This question brings a confused look, but the answer is "YES." My reply will be, "So, let's start to make a difference." My goal here is to make the client feel empowered. Empowering a client will then be a game-changer, following which their outlook on life will change.

Both people and animals can hold emotional baggage in their muscles. There are views on this subject in which some schools view that emotions are stored in the body's fascia. The fascia is a thick layer of connective tissue that surrounds and holds every organ, blood vessel, bone, nerve fibre, and muscle in place. This fantastic structure does far more than provide support because it has nerves, making it almost as sensitive as the skin. Could this be the second brain in the body, and is this what we call our gut feeling? Our gut feeling is what some people call our intuition. Our intuition is powerful, and I believe we have been encouraged to ignore it by people who write textbooks and say that if something can't be proven scientifically, we should not hold that view. What if science and technology were not advanced enough to understand what's happening within and outside the human body? Intuition has been used successfully for thousands of years in every area of the planet and receives more recognition, and I'm sure in time, it will be used more widely.

When we hold emotions in muscles, the muscles can be tight, and this tightness can increase over time and then end up being painful. It's possible that someone may have a niggle in their back, and now and again, it will flare-up. This could be attributed to emotions being held or stuck here. As a therapist, if I can release the tight muscle, the feeling comes up and is released. People will often weep to their heart's content, and when they do, it makes them feel good about releasing whatever they needed to. The release of emotion is an honour to witness, and I always thank the client for their trust.

Someone once asked me if I could treat her husband's back. He had been in pain for a while, and he was continually moaning about his back. They were due to fly off on holiday the next day, and she grumbled that if I couldn't help her husband, it would ruin their holiday. So, I agreed, and later that day, I visited their house. When she opened the door, she confessed that her husband does not believe in complementary therapies and the like. I then went to stand beside this mountain of a man, and his wife announced, "Tony has come to fix your back," to which he looked down at me and said, "Oh, really, if you can help a bit, I'm sure the wife will appreciate it, as she says I'm moaning a lot." I asked him to rank the severity of his pain on a scale of 0 to 10, with 10 being the worst. He described his pain as being at the level of 10.

One look at him, and I could see the pain on his face. As we walked into another room, I could see he could not stand straight or walk without holding his back. I asked him how long he had been suffering, and he turned to me and said, "Oh, about 30 years."

Starting the session, I put my fingers on him, and within a few seconds, he began to cry. The poor man cried hard, and I could do my treatment on him. As I continued, tears rolled down his face, and I could do the work on his back that I needed to. While crying, he revealed all sorts of things that had been on his mind and worried him. When I had finished, I asked him how the pain was, and he looked at me stunned and said it was gone. This change in him made me smile. I then explained that, in my opinion, his continued back issue was because he had been holding his emotional baggage in the muscles at the base of his back. As I released the tightness in those muscles, the emotion was released, which is why he cried. I then congratulated him on letting go of all that emotional stuff and said, "Now it's gone, it doesn't need to come back." He was still astonished that all that pain had completely disappeared.

To me, this is an excellent example of how pain and discomfort are multidimensional and how people can be stuck in a pattern that does not allow the pain to escape.

When I treat people, I think it's essential that the client feels as if someone is listening intently to them. When I have a conversation with a client, I can pick up so much material that can help me formulate a plan of action. How are they describing things? What particular words are they using? Do they understand some of the medical terminologies used by other healthcare professionals?

1. Prevalence of chronic pain in the UK: a systematic review and meta-analysis of population studies. A Fayaz1, P Croft2, R M Langford3, L J Donaldson4, G T Jones5

2. https://www.britishpainsociety.org/mediacentre/news/ british-pain-society-press-release-chronic-pain-costs- the-uk-billions-but-research-funding-is-inadequate/

3. https://www.statista.com/statistics/308201/leading- ten- pets-ranked-by-population-size-in-the-united- kingdom/

3.

What is Complementary Therapy?

People often get confused about the difference between complementary and alternative therapy. Here is how I think about it in my head. I think it's essential to understand the difference between the two; they are not the same and should not be classified as the same.

More and more people are exploring complementary and alternative therapies when they feel that conventional medicine has failed them and they want to know whether anything or what else can be done to help them.

Complementary Therapy

A therapy that can be used alongside any other treatment is given to complement each other and offer the client a better experience and chance of healing. You could combine several therapies or just one, and it all depends on the client's needs at that specific time.

A complementary therapy will not cause any harm and will not replace any medical treatment or advice given to the client.

I can understand why people are sceptical about

complementary or alternative therapies. We have all seen documentaries on TV with people dancing around a tree or drinking some disgusting- looking drinks around a massive fire. A lot of this goes against the treatments we have traditionally seen and experienced through our usual healthcare system.

In the National Health Service, I was a nurse in intensive care at one of the world's leading hospitals. I struggled with the idea of complementary therapies (tree huggers) for years, but this was due to my lack of knowledge. I used to think that modern medicine could be the only thing that worked and that it had robust clinical trials backing up its use or treatment. Complementary and alternative therapies could not work, as they had not been through this level of scrutiny.

Now I look back, realising I was looking at the world with blinkers on and didn't think about the therapies that had been administered for hundreds if not thousands of years with great success.

Why choose complementary therapy?

Many people think about and almost talk themselves out of it because of fear of the unknown.

A complementary therapy should fit in with anything else a client is doing for their health, as it COMPLEMENTS. We shouldn't have to stop or radically change anything else to treat the issue.

I can't guarantee 100% success to a client when treating the issue, but I can give it my best shot. The beautiful thing about the therapy that I use is that I can say that I can't make things worse. We can achieve excellent results by adding something extra to the standard treatment and working with the client, be it a person or an animal.

A vast majority of my clients feel a difference right away. By right away, I mean within a minute of the treatment starting. A confused look on their face demonstrates this, and that makes me smile and giggle. I'm a great one for giggling and laughing. If I can get the clients to think about their bodies and the reactions that are going on and feel a difference, I know changes are starting to happen, and that feels so good to me. When clients concentrate on sensations in their bodies, which could be for days after the treatment has finished, it gives them a feeling of personal responsibility and control over a part of their lives that may have been absent for a while. This personal responsibility and empowerment are compelling in aiding the healing process in my eyes and can help in the recovery of a client's mental and physical health. Depending on the client and the issue, it may not take many sessions to return to normal (whatever normal is for the client).

Alternative Therapy

This type of therapy is given instead of another treatment, and it's an alternative to standard care.

Individualism

Each client I see is an individual, and I feel that they should be treated as such. I have always disliked hearing other healthcare professionals refer to a patient or client by the issue or condition they may have. Suppose you refer to people with the particular issue they have and give them a label of that issue, for example, a right shoulder issue, you will start to treat them all in the same way. Labels are for birthday and Christmas gifts and not clients.

People experience and describe pain differently, so why treat them the same!

I observe the client's body to see if it's out of balance or how they are holding themselves. These are my clues to the issue and to the approach to treating this particular client. This observation is powerful, and if I can relax and use my intuition, I can help a client in their recovery.

4.

What is the EMMETT Technique?

Having broken my back, tried physio, and taken lots of medication that did not work for me and then having acupuncture that changed the spasms in my back made me think long and hard about other therapies and my lack of insight into them.

This encounter fired up my imagination to investigate what other complementary therapies could help me. So, I searched the Internet to see what I could find. Being old and cynical, I thought that if something worked on me, then it did work. I was not really into all this hippy tree-hugging stuff. I researched alternative/complementary therapies. I spent hours and days scouring different websites, articles, and YouTube videos in front of my computer. As weeks went by, I went on a couple of taster days and could not either get on with the therapy or feel comfortable in my back, as I constantly experienced deep burning pain. One therapy I came across was the Australian in origin EMMETT technique. I wasn't able to find much on it, but the one thing that stood out was the claim that a light finger pressure, often over clothes, has instant effects and can cure anybody anywhere. My initial impression was "What a load of utter bollocks." I shut down the computer, and I did not give it any further thought. This thought of thing could not possibly work and its all hocus-pocus.

A few weeks later, again, I was trying to delve into the Internet to find that one particular therapy that could change my life, and I was not having any success. I then came across the EMMETT Technique again and read a little bit more about it. I found out that EMMETT Therapies UK were holding a one-day taster in East Grinstead, which is not that far from where I live, and I thought why not, as I had done a few other taster days. Along I went; there were ten students there, one a physiotherapist, and the rest of us were complete novices at the therapy game. The corrections were demonstrated to us. Then we had to copy what had been shown to us. I could not believe my eyes. I could see people's bodies moving, and they were saying, "Oh, that's nice" and "I feel so much freer." We came to a back correction, and I felt my body move and my back position change. All the students had similar things to say on that day about how they could not understand how fast and easy this was, and the results were terrific. I drove home convinced that the instructor had hypnotised us, and that's why we all felt different and had less pain. Now I know it was a load of bollocks. That evening I had to sort out my head and prove we had been hypnotised, so I went back to the Internet to look at group hypnosis, and frustratingly, I could not find out how this instructor had done it to us. The following day, I got out of bed more manageable than I had done in months. Now I was thinking, "Oh bugger, there might be something in this after all, and it might not be the scam I thought it was."

After the taster session although my back pain was so much better, and on some days, I would say it was a niggle more than a pain, I convinced myself that it was just natural healing that had taken place and nothing else. I then dismissed everything that had happened on the EMMETT training day and got on with life as usual.

A month or so later, I picked up a copy of Horse and Hound and saw an advert for a course on using the EMMETT technique on horses. This course was an excellent opportunity for me to finally prove to myself properly that the EMMETT technique was, in my view, a load of bollocks. I thought you couldn't get a placebo effect on a horse, so if I saw something change, it had to be a result of the intervention I had just done. So, I signed up for the course with two instructors who flew over from Australia to teach it.

Day one of the course dawned, and I felt like a fish out of water, as I was the only person in the group that was not already a horse therapist of some description. We went to work on the horses, and, in my mind, this was going to be the proof I needed. When this therapy didn't work, I could walk away, proving the point to myself. The first mare I had to work on had her owner standing there, watching the new technique being used on her baby. As I approached the mare, she turned her head, bared her teeth, and raised her hip as if she would kick out. The owner smiled like a Cheshire Cat as she did this, and I thought, "Oh great, she knows I'm either going to get bitten or kicked." I planned that I would say, "Oh, it's ok, I'm not hurt," as the mare exacted her revenge for having to be with us and not in the field with her mates.

I approached the mare and said, "Hello." I didn't waste any time and swooped in, doing the first correction, and she turned her head and started licking my arm, much to my surprise. The owner walked away. We then received feedback on our performance from the instructors, and all the students gave our feedback on what results we saw. We then stopped for a coffee break, and the owner of the mare I had been working with came over, and I said how nice it was to have her mare lick my arm as if to say, thank you. Well, I was shocked at the response of that woman: "That bitch hasn't done that to me in the ten years I've had her." To me, that was it. This bloody stuff did work, after all. The more treatment this horse had for the rest of the day, the more she wanted a cuddle, and she was so loving. I went home thinking that now I had to look at things differently. This day had been a real game-changer for me.

Day two of the course and standing in the yard was the owner and her mare that I had worked on the day before. As we got closer, she said that she had ridden the mare last evening, the nicest ride she had ever had, and if we wanted, we could use her mare again. This feedback was the icing on the cake for me. Not only did we see the mare's body and nature change the day before, but the rider noticed it as well. I was then sold on this strange therapy from that moment.

I signed up for the rest of the course. A part of the horse course also teaches how to treat the rider, and as it was the same corrections I had learned on the one-day taster day, with practice, I felt confident at using them. When I tried these corrections on friends, they all said how nice they were and how much more comfortable they felt. This positive feedback led me to investigate and sign up for the EMMETT course on people (where was this going to lead me!).

I started the course for people and felt even more out of place as I was the only person who was not already an established therapist. During the introductions around the room, I felt somewhat inadequate. Doing this course was an anxious time for me. I had to give feedback to the instructor about what we felt and noticed when doing the corrections. Some people could feel energetic changes and the energy run down the body being treated and left through the little toe. That technical term was in my head again. "Oh, bollocks. what were they seeing!?" I couldn't see anything except that the foot was still at the bottom of the leg. I mentioned to the instructor that I thought that this form of EMMETT was not for me. She asked me why, and I explained how I couldn't feel or see what everyone else was feeling and seeing and that I questioned whether I was doing everything right. Her reply was not to notice what other people were saying, as some people were saying those things to make themselves feel better, and that it was their ego getting in the way. I went home and slept on it and returned for day two of the course, and that morning, I did a correction on someone, and the body pushed me off with the power of the muscle release. Well, I was shocked by what the hell happened there! I looked over, and the instructor just smiled back at me, as she knew something had just happened by the look on my face.

I completed the training in both horses and people and started to enjoy myself and believe that my possibilities from this therapy were endless.

I started doing treatments every weekend and during my holidays from work. Each time, I received terrific feedback from people, and the more I treated, the more I wanted to. As much as I loved this work, I had to separate it from my day job. At the time, I worked in the NHS as a matron in adult intensive care, specialising in research and a specific type of life-support machine (high-frequency ventilation). I had at that time been working in that environment for over 20 years. I wondered that if people found out I was a complementary therapist, would they call me a "Tree Hugger" or "Hippy"? Eventually, people, especially the nurses, started to find out through social media that I was doing complementary therapy. Some of them asked me what this EMMETT stuff was, so that was my opportunity to jump into action. "Let me show you" was the stock answer to the question.

As I'm sure you know, nurses are notorious for having back and neck issues. Well, I could make them feel better within a couple of minutes. It was a beautiful experience, and they loved it. Some had had pain for years and had unsuccessfully tried all sorts of remedies, and then I came along with the lightest of pressure, and the pain was gone. After a while, nurses used to turn up at my office door and ask, "Can you sort my back out, please?" and their issues were sorted in no time at all.

One particular day, a medical consultant I was working with asked me what on earth was I doing as I was treating nurses backs in the middle of the intensive care unit. For years, this man had suffered from a bad neck issue, so he was the ideal candidate for a quick treatment/demonstration. I performed the correction, and his neck straightened up for the first time in years. He looked at me and remarked, "How the hell have you done that? And remember who my wife is." His wife was a consultant physiotherapist, who had been treating him for years and had even used acupuncture. They had never obtained the result I did within two minutes. After some thought, I asked him whether I could offer the treatment out to the staff in the department as I was sure it would help. We agreed it would be a nice thing to offer. For three months, I provided the treatments to all department staff (1,200 of them). I completed a data recording exercise of the people I had treated, so we could conduct an evaluation.

I used to have consultant anaesthetists at my door at 8 am for me to treat their backs before they started a long list in the operating rooms. We had people who were on long-term sick leave with back issues come and see me once, and they were then reassessed by occupational health and allowed back to work. I have since published this data, and it shows that the EMMETT technique effectively treats back pain significantly.

When this was going on, Ross Emmett the founder of the technique, had been in England and had asked me if I would like to become the senior instructor for his animal courses in the UK and Ireland. It was a message from the gods. I had worked in the NHS for so long I would leave and have a small pension and then top it up with a bit of therapy work, so I jumped at the invitation.

I think back now and realise I must have been dreaming when I felt that I could be out on my horse two or three days a week enjoying the semi-retired life. Well, that's never happened.

The EMMETT technique is Ross Emmett's work, a highly gifted bodywork therapist based in Townsville, Queensland, Australia.

Who is Ross Emmett?

Ross is an Australian born in Tasmania in December 1945 and is the eldest of five children. He was the sort of child that was always in trouble at school. Ross is dyslexic, and that was not even on anyone's radar in those days. So, to hide this, he became the class clown, and his mother said he suffered from "Little Bugger Syndrome" because he was always in trouble. However, this dyslexia has allowed Ross to see things differently, and I see it as a tremendous gift that he has.

The EMMETT technique first evolved as a means for Ross to treat sick and distressed animals. He has always cared for animals and their well-being. His experience working as an animal attendant in a research facility, an Australian Dog Obedience Judge, and a successful animal trainer has helped him gain unique insights into the development of this method. Ross discovered that the technique worked as effectively on the handlers as it did on their animals.

Working in bodywork as a massage and remedial therapist running busy clinical practices in Mt Isa (1981–1999) and Townsville (1999–2008), Australia, allowed Ross to develop the technique further. What initially began as a massage business in Mount Isa in the early 1980s soon allowed him to develop a reputation for making his clients get fast, effective results. His busy Mount Isa practice treated, on average, 100 people per week.

Due to his location in the Australian Outback, his clientele over the years were often people from cattle stations and mines situated hundreds of kilometres away. They had limited access to therapy and little time for treatment. The visit to town needed to provide both instant relief and lasting comfort due to their inability to receive follow-up treatments.

In 1983, Ross began teaching massage therapy and has, since then, trained people in many other modalities, including Bowen therapy. Through the support of other practitioners, particularly the encouragement of a Townsville doctor, he started teaching his technique, commonly known now as the EMMETT technique. It is now taught in 40 countries worldwide.

5.

How Does EMMETT Work?

How EMMETT works is a question I get asked the most, usually after the client demands, "How the hell did you do that?"

From what we can work out so far, it's believed that a light touch on the skin triggers a neurological response between the brain and the soft tissues we work on. This touch at specific points is almost as if pressing a reset button that resets the muscle memory. Making the muscle relax releases the built-up tension and produces a movement restriction.

The touch is almost as light as when you try to pick a butterfly up by its wings. It's that gentle. Yet if the body that's being treated wants more pressure, it leans into you and increases the tension.

Animals respond to the light pressure exceptionally well, which they find pleasant and relaxing. It also transforms the bond between myself and the animal very quickly, and a typical response from an owner is, "Oh, they don't usually do that to strangers." Animals are compassionate beings, and I see treatment as working together in the time required for the animal. When an animal is processing what I have just done, sometimes they go into a trance-like state, and they look so serene and happy.

You see, I understand that all muscles have a memory. They know where they should be and work when the body is balanced, and everything is fine. But when the body is imbalanced or injured, the muscles have to compensate, creating a false memory. This false muscle memory is how we survive. Otherwise, life would grind to a halt with every injury. We have to carry on with life, and we constantly think that given some time and a few painkillers, everything will be back to normal in no time. That is not always the case. The pain does not go away, and we try to ignore it and put it in the back of our minds.

Another way of looking at how this therapy works is to imagine a touch screen. In this day and age, we are all used to them. Touch the screen lightly, and the app or program opens up. Touch the screen too hard or in the wrong place, and nothing happens. Touch it for too long, and it goes into a meltdown, and nothing knows how to work.

We believe that the points we use for this technique are the sensory receptors (buttons). When they are activated appropriately, a communication with the brain generates a corresponding relaxation response.

There are specific receptors all over the body, and

connecting the points in a certain way creates an immediate response. I get a distinct look when this happens to a client, and it does not matter whether it's a person or an animal. It's the look of utter amazement or "What the hell have you just done!" When I see this reaction, I giggle or laugh. I'm a great one for laughing anyway. Sometimes a client will say, "You are always giggling or laughing." It's simply because I can feel things starting to change under my fingers, and I know the client has not registered it yet. Then BOOM, it happens, and the muscle moves, and I get the look.

Ross Emmett once explained to me that nobody knows how his technique works at this moment in time. One day technology will catch up, and we will then start to understand its mechanism. Today, a few fragments of scientific work are being done.

For me, one of the great things about this technique is that it's all done as gently as possible, and we are not out to cause pain. The old saying of "No pain, no gain" is not in our vocabulary, which is also my personal belief. I went to a physio many years ago with a neck issue, and the pressure she was applying on my neck was so painful I was screaming for her to stop. She told me to man up and take the pain, as it would do me good, and that she had to create pain, which would initiate action in my neck to solve my issue. Then, I didn't know any better and vowed never to return to her again and pay for the privilege. As she was inflicting the treatment on me, I was scared that she would break my neck or cause permanent damage. That experience taught me a good lesson. Don't Hurt People or Animals. If I had hurt a patient in my old NHS job, I would have been horrified and even disciplined for it.

Additionally, when I had my significant back injury, I went to an osteopath, and he kept cracking my back. I wasn't too fond of it, and after a few sessions, when there was no change for me, I decided to try another therapy.

After a couple of years, I reflected on both treatments I have just mentioned. I realised that if I knew these treatment sessions would hurt or scare me, how could I relax properly, allowing my body to respond to the treatments on me! In my mind, that would almost be counterproductive to healing my issues.

While we are on the subject of using light pressure, I must admit that, to some people, it seems odd. These people are used to therapists using lots of pressure and sometimes so much pressure that they leave a bruise. Using lots of pressure on clients, some therapists start having wrist and shoulder issues, limiting their working life. Since I have been teaching the technique on horses and dogs, I have trained semi-retired therapists, and using a light touch, they can carry on working in an area they love. As they no longer use the amount of pressure they were using previously, their health has improved. Now, to me, this is a beautiful thing.

Looking back at this chapter, you can see that this technique is non-invasive, gentle, and straightforward to administer.

6.

Animals Are So Much Easier to Treat

<hr>

I have been an animal lover and a horse and dog owner for years. When I saw the behaviour of the horse change on my first EMMETT animal course, it changed my life path. Treating animals is rewarding and satisfying when you hear from the owner how different the animal is following their treatment. A horse revealed to me the truth about this technique and its power, and for that, I am grateful.

When I talk about animals, I am referring mainly to horses and dogs, as they have taught me so much since I started listening to them while helping them with my EMMETT skills. One of the reasons is that people have so much in their heads that gets in the way, while animals do not. They often sense why I am there when I meet them and offer me the part of their body they need me to work on.

Animals can also share powerful bonds with their owners. It's not uncommon to see someone walking their dog, and both the owner and dog have the same limp. The bond can be that strong. A vet once told me that when he sees a new dog for the first time, he likes to ask the owner what medical problems they have, and then he knows where to start with the dog.

We can use dogs to detect if someone has an epileptic fit or their blood sugar has gone too low. Dogs can feel if the owner is unwell, and they then try to comfort the owner. Dogs are used to assisting people with mental health issues, and the dog knows when a person needs more attention without being told. If we knew everything that animals could feel and sense, it would blow our minds.

Animals express their pain or discomfort very differently from humans. There could be a change in how they walk or run, often slower, limping, and head nodding as they walk or trot. You may even notice changes to their posture or unexplained personality changes, generally being more "grumpy." Sometimes, if they have been trying to tell people about the problem and people are not listening, the animal can get frustrated. The animal then tries to show the people more expressively, and often this is classified as a behavioural issue. If you kept telling people you were in pain, and nobody listened or offered to help, I'm sure you would get grumpy as well (I know I would).

When I walk into a stable, it's not unusual for a horse to move towards me and stop with the part of the body they want me to treat right in front of me. I smile when this happens and just do as the animal tells me. It could be a dog that does not let me leave until I have done more work with them. I find this part of my work exciting and amusing. Animals do not hang around if they are not benefitting from the interaction, and when the owners see this happening, they know the animal is enjoying itself.

When treating an animal, I often have to treat the dog owner/ caregiver or the horse and rider. It's a question of balance. If the dog has a tight shoulder and neck, a strong possibility is that the dog pulls on the lead, which impacts the person at the other end of the leash.

If I treat just the dog, I'm only doing half a job, so while the dog is processing the work I have just done, I take that opportunity to treat the person. Processing is when the animal appears relaxed and can look as if they have been sedated. This deep relaxation allows the body and mind to reset. It has been suggested that the brain goes into a deeply relaxed state, which could be the same as meditating, allowing the body to repair itself. When I treat people, they often sit down after I have left and fall asleep, allowing this processing to occur.

Should it be a horse I'm treating, I will look at the rider. If they are not balanced, they will be sitting in the saddle like the leaning tower of Pisa. I have on many occasions treated the rider while in the saddle. I love doing this. When I'm correcting the rider, I can see the horse change, and then they turn and look at me with that look!

Churchill's Story

I was once asked to treat a tortoise. Yes, your eyes are not deceiving you, a tortoise. It lived in a rescue centre and was part of the tortoise's 100th birthday celebrations, in which it had lots of publicity photos taken. This tortoise had survived the Second World War blitz and was called Churchill. However, when Churchill was 60 years old, they found out that Churchill was a girl.

So, on the day the keeper handed me Churchill, I was amazed that she was pretty relaxed. As soon as I started treating her through her shell, she relaxed further, and her head and legs allowed me to get my fingers just under the shell.

I did a few corrections and placed her on the ground when I finished. She stayed still for a few seconds and then walked over to a bush and planted herself on the ground with her head under the bush. She was there for about five minutes and then suddenly turned around, and she was off as if she was in a race. Her keeper laughed and said he had never seen her move so fast in all the years he had cared for her.

Amelia's Story

Amelia was a cow that a vet had seen following a suspected fall in a field. She was six months pregnant and unable to stand up or walk. The vet assessed her and opined that nothing could be done to help her, and the best plan would be to put her to sleep. Not doing anything was not an option for the farmer and his family, as they thought the cow deserved more. They started her on a homeopathic preparation to help with swelling and bruising and gave her plenty of rest in a nice warm pen. After a week or so, she managed to stand up and walk with extreme difficulty. I was asked if I could help, which, of course, I said I believed I could. This farmer's daughter had heard of my working on a couple of cows on another farm, and they had responded well to my treatment.

Off I went and was introduced to this amazing cow who seemed to understand why I was there, although she was nervous about meeting me. She tried to walk away from me and really struggled. I did my best to let her know that I was not a vet and would not inject her (she is wary of vets). I made my first move, and she looked at me as if saying, "What the hell was that!" She stood still, completely mesmerised. The farmer's wife and daughter who were watching me looked puzzled. I love this look, and when it happens, I'm jumping up and down inside as I then know something is changing in the body I'm treating. Amelia was in a trance for a few minutes, and when she came back into the room, she lay down on the nice straw bed and lifted her leg for me to treat. So, I knelt beside her and worked on her leg. She was so gentle, and it was a privilege working with her.

Of course, the weight of that massive baby inside her would slow down the healing. As the baby grew, it could also cause issues for her. The day after my visit, I received a text message to say she was standing much more comfortably and walking better.

I returned a week later, and as soon as she saw me, Amelia once more lay down for me to work on her. After a while, she stood up and turned around so that I could work on her other leg. She was licking me, and every time I took my fingers off her, she very gently touched me with her nose as if to say thank you.

After another couple of treatments, she was able to move around so much better, but the baby's weight prevented the completion of the healing process. It was then a waiting game for the birth to ease the weight on the leg from the position the baby was laying inside her.

A few weeks later, I received a text saying that Amelia had given birth and that they were both fine. I couldn't wait to see them. As soon as I got to the pen, Amelia came over to say hello and nudged her baby towards me as if she was introducing us. I treated her, and I felt significant changes in her back, hips, and legs. Less than a month later, she was out in the fields with the rest of the herd, and you would not know she had ever had anything wrong with her.

Jake's Story

Jake was a Great Dane and a complete gentleman. He had been diagnosed with an incurable progressive neurological condition. He could be walking along, and his back end would go from underneath him, and he would fall over. This condition affected him both physically and mentally and knocked out his confidence. Additionally, if he fell over, it would take at least two people to lift him again with his size.

I went to see him and ended up sitting in his bed with him. I took my time to do everything I needed to do at his pace. His owner/caregiver watched his reaction and could tell that he enjoyed having his therapist sitting in his bed with him and making him feel good. The next day, I received a message that he had been running around and playing in his afternoon walk, which he had not done in months.

Over the next 18 months, I went to see him regularly to keep his body as comfortable as possible and support him. Whenever he saw me, he would bark as if saying, "Where have you been?" This made me smile so much. If he were in his bed, he would roll onto his back, and we needed to have some fuss and a cuddle before we got down to some work.

If, however, he was in the garden, he would be sitting there like the lord of the manor and as if he owned the place and we were there just to serve him.

He would also not let me leave until he had finished with me. If I went to stand up, he would soon tell me that I was not going. He would put one of his giant paws on me or his head.

How could I not do as my client wanted! We built such a great friendship, and I loved being around him.

The last time I saw Jake was on an afternoon, when he was sitting in the garden under a gazebo in the brilliant sunshine like the true gent he was.

He had an excellent session, and as I was treating him, various family members came and sat with us. They were all there sitting around us by the time I had finished, and Jake loved it. He was so content, and again, if I said it was time to go or tried to get up, he stopped me. So, I stayed and enjoyed the sunshine with them all.

Two days later, I got a message saying that Jake had passed away from a stroke. I immediately thought of that beautiful afternoon and cried for my friend. When I go to the house where he lived, I can still feel him and expect him to come looking for me.

Can You Treat Our Rabbit, Please?

Once, I arrived at a clients' house to treat his chronic back pain issues. The usual thing that happened when I came was that the two large dogs were very excited to see me and insisted I treat them first before their owner. The dogs made it known to both myself and their owner that I was there to see them first. They would not let their owner come anywhere near me.

Once I had done a couple of bits on them, they would sit and watch me work on their Dad. I could see in their faces how they were both reacting to the work I was doing with their Dad, and that can happen when there is a strong bond between owner and animal.

Anyway, as I reached the end of the session, the chap asked me, "Could you treat one of my wife's rabbits, please?" It seems just before I arrived at the house for the appointment the rabbit had been excited to be let out of her hutch to play with her best friend (one of the dogs).

As the hutch door opened, she jumped out as usual onto the dog's back. But this time, she slipped and landed on her neck and shoulder; ever since she could not hold her head straight.

So off we went to see her, and as I held her in my arms, I had an audience of the dog owner and his wife and the two dogs watching me. I did one correction on the rabbit, and one of the dogs jumped up as the rabbit shook. I laid the rabbit on the ground, and off she went chasing the dogs with a straight- looking neck and darting at such speed that it was clear she was not in any pain.

On a day like that, how could I not enjoy where my life had gone!

7.

Self-Care

What is self-care? To me, it seems a strange thing. To care for yourself! What's all that about?

From what I can tell, most people choose a caring profession because, to some degree, they need caring for themselves but don't want to dig deep to find the issue. It's easier to find someone else to care for. Caring for others is something I did for years and years in my nursing career. The patient always came first, and it made me forget myself. Putting everyone else first can become a habit, and after a while, you can forget who you are. Not caring for yourself can eventually take its toll on both your body and mind. How can you carry on giving your best when the batteries are empty? To give my best while working, I have found that I need to think about and care for myself to keep my batteries full and my mind free of clutter to let me concentrate on the job at hand.

I have started to meditate (it sounds easier than it is to practice) and have been exploring different meditation types that suit me and my lifestyle. When I get it right, it feels beautiful and rejuvenating. I'm delving into an exploration of my health that I possibly would have laughed at a few years ago.

One of the great qualities of the EMMET technique is that there is so much of it that you can do for yourself. You need to be taught these things in an EMMETT course, and there are now several different courses (Pilates instructors, mother and baby, midwifery, foot specialist, to name a few). Simply watching a YouTube video or reading instructions, you will miss things. There is much more to EMMETT than just the light pressure. It's about the direction of the finger/pressure, it's duration, and the signs the body gives you that something is happening. Just like anything else, if it's not executed properly, it won't work. Learning from an instructor or tutor of the technique helps preserve the technique's integrity and maintains standards. If just anyone could teach the technique, it would be like a game of Chinese whispers and the magic of the therapy would be lost. An interpretation of another complementary therapy has already happened, and it ruined the therapy by not delivering the treatment as it should be.

Suppose there is one particular correction vital to the body being treated; an EMMETT therapist will often teach the parent, partner, owner, and caregiver how to do the correction. Teaching a particular correction empowers and helps everyone involved.

One aspect of my vocation is travelling all over the UK and Ireland, demonstrating this technique on horses and dogs. I do an awful lot of mileage in my car. I have been caught by people releasing my neck when I'm sitting at traffic lights. But it takes me seconds to release the muscles, and it feels so good although sometimes I get funny looks from people at traffic lights when they see me!

I think it's such a great gift we can pass on to people. Ross Emmett, the founder of the technique, has put together a one- day course for anyone to attend, and it teaches people how to use the technique on family and friends.

When the COVID lockdowns first happened, Ross generously shared a little sequence of his work called "Recovery". It's a sequence of seven small moves that can relieve anyone or any animal experiencing deep anxiety or distress. For legal reasons, I can't put the instructions on how to do this into my book. But if you want to know more, don't hesitate to get in touch with me, and I will point you in the right direction for video's that explains much more than you can find on paper.

I have taught this technique to so many people, and their feedback after using this little sequence is incredible. Parents have used it on their children to calm them down, and animal owners have used it on their anxious pets. They all say the same things afterwards, "That stuff is amazing, and it worked so quickly.".

8.

My Personal Experience with Emmett
(Mike Warren)

In April 2015, I was struck down suddenly by an illness that left me paralysed I was taken to three different hospitals before they identified my condition as amyloidosis. Altogether, I spent eight months away from home utterly dependent on the nurses to help me in every way. I had three rounds of chemotherapy because I was also diagnosed with multiple myeloma. During my stay in the hospital, I also saw some neuro physiotherapists, who tried to make me able to move again. It was challenging and complicated, as I also suffered from incredibly debilitating pain. I took so many painkilling drugs that I felt as if in a permanent haze. Before I came home, the doctors had given me up to two years to live. They also said it was unlikely that I would walk again. All this negativity resulted in me feeling very depressed and really in a bad place mentally.

Even after returning home in about 4–5 months, my pain and physical health had not improved. I had lost over eight stone in weight, resulting in my not having the muscle power to do much. Then my partner told me about a Facebook friend doing alternative work with horses and dogs. He told me he had messaged him and said he would come and see me. I objected, as I didn't believe in mumbo jumbo. Thankfully, he took no notice of my objections, which is why Tony Sherry ultimately came to see me.

Initially, we chatted, and then Tony started putting his fingers on my legs. I couldn't feel anything at all, but I did notice a slightly warm feeling, and my mind told me it was all imagination. Tony spent about 30 minutes doing his stuff. I was glad when he stopped. I did enjoy the stories Tony relayed about the animals he had treated, but again, to be honest, I thought them to be a bit far-fetched. When he had left, I told my partner that I didn't want him coming to see me again. However, he (thankfully) did not heed me, as Tony came to see me again a few days later. Once again, he worked on my legs, while I kept thinking it was a waste of time. During the next few hours, I did think that the pain was easing a bit, but I still didn't think it was anything to do with the therapy. After a few more sessions, I noticed the pain had decreased, and I could move my legs and feet a little. I then began to think that it may be the Emmett that was helping. I still had no feeling in my lower body, but I also did not experience the pain I had had in my legs. For a few months, Tony worked on my legs until the point came at which I reduced my painkillers considerably.

I was still seeing the neuro physiotherapist but was not getting on too well with the exercises. I also had no natural feeling in my hands, and I couldn't hold a pen or knife and fork, etc. I couldn't raise my arms at all. One day, I told Tony about the physiotherapist's attempts to get my arms moving, and he said he could help. He made one finger move on my shoulders, and it felt like a miracle. I could raise my arms over my head without any pain at all. This action convinced me that Emmett was a revolutionary addition to the medical profession.

As time went by, the sensation in my hands improved, and I was also able to stand up with the help of a walking frame. As I spent more time with Tony, I found I could do more and more. Eventually, I started to take a step or two and began to feel my feet and legs a bit. Tony, with his moves, helped my body start work. After about six months, I stopped taking any painkillers. I stopped the chemotherapy as it made me very sick and giddy. My blood pressure had been very low, which began to improve slightly. I continued to have the therapy, and we started to set goals such as standing with a stick and then walking with it. I began to gain strength and put on weight. As soon as my muscles improved, I was able to move better. Emmett helped me in so many ways, and I can now walk with the aid of sticks and stand without any support. We are currently working on my balance and getting my nerves to recognise different parts of my body. I think it is essential to remember that the doctors had told me that I would not be able to walk again, but today I can walk, albeit with a stick, and use my arms and hands. The sensations are coming back in my feet and legs.

I believe that Emmett should be available to many more people, and after the complete surprise and incredulity my doctor showed when he saw me stand and walk, I trust the NHS will look at this treatment. Emmett has given me a life that can considerably help many others. I can only thank Tony and Emmett for all of this. I shudder to think what I may have been like if I hadn't met Tony - Many, many thanks.

My Experience of Treating Mike Warren (Tony Sherry)

A friend asked me if I could help his partner, who was suffering from a neurological condition (amyloidosis) and was in a lot of pain. I, of course, said that I believed I could.

My first impression of meeting Mike was of a man who was in far more pain than he was letting on, and his mind was in a very dark place. He was dependent on his partner/carer and carers coming in to help with all personal care, etc. This life-changing condition had completely devastated Mike and everyone around him.

Mike was in so much pain he was reluctant to move, and moving his knees had to be completed in a slow and controlled way to reduce the pain. I could see on his face the extreme amount of pain he was experiencing with every movement. He told me the story of his illness – what had happened to him, and how he had got to this point in his life.

The main aim of my first treatment was to try and reduce the pain in his legs. The moment I put my fingers on his cold legs, I could feel the muscles moving under my fingertips. I could see by Mike's reaction that he could not feel what I was doing. As Mike was a farmer and had been so his whole life before he became ill, I spoke about the animals I had treated, which took his focus away from the pain. After a few treatments, I could touch Mike' feet, and his toes started to move, much to his surprise. At the same time, he mentioned how tight his shoulders felt, and he could not raise his arms. I put my finger on his shoulder and completed a quick EMMETT move, and told him to raise his arms. Mike looked at me as if I was barmy, as he had just said he could not move them. He started to raise his arms, and his face was a picture because his arms kept going up, and then he began to wave them around, saying, "But you hardly touched me," and they have stayed free ever since. Treating his forearms changed the feeling in his fingers so much that he could start to hold a proper cup (not a plastic beaker) and use cutlery.

Over a few weeks, we started to see more movement in Mike's feet and legs. As the changes happened, Mike reduced his painkilling medication and was not taking any before long. This significantly affected his mental health, and I could begin to see a different man in front of me. The change in his muscles has been an interesting one to see and treat; due to his medical condition, the neural pathway is not intact or predictable. Using the EMMETT technique principles, I have been amazed at the changes in these paralysed legs. Treatment sessions typically last much longer than that of my usual clients. The treatments can also be amusing because when working on Mike's feet, his thighs react, and the twitches in the muscles are visible and will go on for minutes after my fingers have come off.

The muscles reacting so well to the treatments have had a knock- on effect on his heart, and his blood pressure is now much better than it has been since he was taken ill.

Over the past couple of months, if I am away teaching EMMETT4Animals, Mike receives an EMMETT treatment from his partner. Mike was pleased to tell me that he has the same reaction to his treatments when John treats him as when I do.

We have now got to the point where Mike can move his ankles and feel me touch the bottom of his feet. If I tickle his left foot, he jumps, and now the feeling is coming back into his right foot. Mike can now get up from his chair and stand unaided without holding onto anything. His balance improves on each visit, and he can stand much straighter. If he uses two ski sticks, he can walk in a more upright position and sports a big smile on his face.

Persistence and a positive attitude from myself have paid off.

How Mike's Partner has viewed his treatment with me

My name is Gary Roberts, and I am the partner of Mike Warren, whom Tony has been treating for the past 2—3 years. Mike fell ill with amyloidosis and multiple myeloma in early 2015, and he became paralysed almost overnight. After being in hospital for eight months, he was discharged home under palliative care. He could not walk or move his arms properly and was in significant neurological pain. He refused to continue his chemotherapy, and I was apprehensive about his outcome. I was looking through some of my Facebook friends, and I saw that Tony was doing something called EMMETT therapy. I contacted him and arranged for him to see Mike.

The first couple of times, Mike did not seem convinced that the therapy was doing any good, and I persuaded him to continue, and he began to find that the terrible pain started to settle. After approximately three months, he discontinued his painkillers and was able to stand with the help of a frame for a few minutes. His hands and arms were very stiff, and Tony worked on them, and Mike was able to raise his arms and grip with his hands. As time passed, Mike could walk with the aid of a frame, and after about a year, he walked a few steps with a walking stick.

From my point of view, I found someone in Tony, who I could talk with about my concerns and try to take some positives out of something very negative. Tony helped me to dream of a future where I thought there was none. His cheery attitude was invaluable, especially as I felt confronted by very negative doctors who only gave me little hope of recovery. I'm not sure I would have coped without Tony's encouragement, primarily his positive actions and attitude toward Mike.

EMMETT has worked miracles, as I thought along with the doctors that Mike would never walk, or come to that, survive. He continues to receive EMMETT, and it has transformed our lives. I don't think Mike would be here without Tony's care, and I can only thank him most sincerely for that.

9.

Conclusion

I believe that pain should not necessarily be a part of anyone's life or future, and being pain-free should be for both people and animals.

If you are suffering from pain, please don't give up; if you meet a health professional that says, "There is nothing that can be done to help you, you will just have to live with it," the answer to that is, "No, you don't." Look at me and the manner in which I found my way out of that horrible place. Don't let it wear you down and take its toll on you because it often does without you realising it. When you suffer, so do your loved ones. Working alongside a complementary therapist, you will find that loads can be done to help. We don't need to learn how to live with pain.

Self-care is very important for everyone, and it's never too late to start. Taking regular time for yourself will help manage any pain, even if it's 15 minutes, three times a week to begin with. You could read a book or do something that you enjoy, and helping to maintain yourself will affect others around you.

Thank you for reading my book. I hope you now have a

better insight into who I am, what I stand for, and what is my journey with pain. You can say that the pain I experienced changed my life for the better. Animals showed me how the powerful therapy I use works so well. I love what I'm doing and believe that my life has led to this point.

Now that you have got this far, why don't you contact me and discuss how I can help you or someone you know?

What Next?

I want to promote the technique and introduce it into the NHS as I believe it would benefit so many people and could potentially save so much time and money. My GP is interested in discussing how I can take EMMETT into the surgery and assist their patients. Nursing and medical staff could take the EMMETT technique to so many areas to enhance their working lives and that of their patients.

I would also like to see EMMETT practiced in animal rescue centres. Using the technique in such places would help so many animals overcome emotional difficulties and help them find the best forever home.

I would also like to research more into the effectiveness of the technique.

I want my business to expand and have a great team of people working with me to improve the quality of life for anyone experiencing pain or a movement restriction.

If you are reading this book, please help me spread the word, and together, we can improve the lives of both people and animals.

Testimonials

———◦◦◦———

Dear Tony,

Thank you for seeing me and helping to resolve the pain.

I had a knee injury six years ago, had surgery, and was on crutches for over a year. I had lived with this pain and had been taking very strong pain killers with very little effect and many side effects. This limited my activities. I couldn't climb stairs. Alighting stairs was excruciatingly painful. I had spent so much money on many therapies with very little effect.

By chance, I met you and found out about your therapy, the Emmett technique. I wasn't sure what you do or what the treatment entailed.

When you gently touched the affected area, I was under the impression that you were just assessing my knee. You asked me to walk a short distance from my sitting position and back to you, which I thought was part of the assessment.

To my amazement, my pain suddenly disappeared, which I didn't understand.

I didn't believe that it was real, I thought it might all come back again. That night, I had the most peaceful and pain-free sleep in many years.

The pain, tightness, and swelling had completely disappeared. I still can't believe it and keep expecting it to come back, but nothing has happened since and it has been about six months.

I sing your praises to everyone I meet, as I couldn't believe what looks like a simple touch could have such a positive impact on my life, which is now painkiller-free and pain-free.

Thank you, Tony, I wish I had known about your technique sooner. Aminata

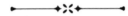

Dear Tony,

Thank you very much for seeing me and letting me try Emmet therapy.

I had shoulder pains for ten years. Occasionally, this pain was aggravated by bad posture and lifting objects. My pain score was 6/10, limiting my range of motion and occasionally triggering stress headache.

I saw Tony for a meeting one time, and at that time, I was in pain. He asked me if I would like to try Emmet therapy. I thought he was joking when he told me about the concept. I was a bit sceptical then, but the only way to know this worked was to try it. I used a TENS machine occasionally – TENS works, but you need to have it on for at least 3–4 hrs.

When Tony touched my shoulder (I barely felt it), the pain instantly disappeared. I was surprised by my reaction. I cried! The feeling of an instant disappearance of a niggling pain was exhilarating! And it was like a miracle because I did not even feel any sensation during the therapy (i.e., touch, pressure at the point of pain, etc.).

I recommend this therapy, especially, if you have an acute episode of pain.

Thanks, Tony. Roy

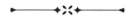

Hi everyone,

I was recommended Emmett therapy after having serious left leg pain for nearly two years. Medical investigations failed to pinpoint the cause of pain. I was in agony during my first visit to Tony. I couldn't bend my left leg when I was sitting down. I couldn't do stairs and my walking was affected.

When I saw Tony, he acted professionally and explained everything to me beforehand. He then used light pressure at points on the affected leg and then asked me to walk around. I could feel that my walking was better; however, the pain remained. Tony reassured me that I should feel a lot better in a few days. As days went by, I continued to get better and better, and now I can do 12-floor stairs, run on the treadmill for half an hour, and sit with a bent knee with ease. Thanks to

Tony.

Jane

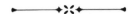

One of my Liveries sent me a message. Some chap in Kent was looking for a yard in Norfolk to run a therapy course. I got in touch and offered our yard but didn't think much of it.

This chap, Tony Sherry, came up to look around and discuss the course. I have to say that my ears pricked up when I heard what the course entailed, but I was sceptical. It sounded far too good to be true!

Then, I got asked if I could host a session for the trainers. Someone from Australia was coming over, and the trainers wanted to get together. Fair enough, after all, the ponies would get free treatment. That way I could see what it involved.

The day arrived, as did Tony. Unfortunately, I had pulled my back the day before and could barely move! Tony smiled and asked where it hurt. I gingerly motioned to the worst bit. Seconds later, the pain had gone! He then set about re-centring my centre of gravity?!? Now I was getting interested!

The trainers arrived, and I introduced them to my horse. I had been with her for over 11 years. I knew her and she knew me! I used her first as I can easily tell whether something is genuinely working or it is just a gimmick. You can imagine my surprise (and disbelief!) when my back started to tingle. I was trying to muck out while keeping an eye on my horse. I kept stopping to try and work out what I was feeling. Then Neil, the Australian, turned and asked how well I knew the horse. I told him how long I had had her and he smiled. He told me which parts of my neck and back would be 'tingling', and said that they were the releases he had just done on my horse.

No way! It was not possible! He smiled and then Tony did something to her…and I nearly lost my balance! Apparently, that was the same thing they had just done to my horse? And she was looking just as puzzled as I was!

Fast forward to today…

I've qualified in both the horse and people courses. Thanks to Tony, I have been able to make the horses I ride more supple than I have ever known them. I have been able to release tension in the horses I coach within 15 minutes, when before it would have taken at least six months of hard work. I have learned (Let's be honest, I'm still getting my head around it!) the possibilities of this developing therapy.

He has given me a glimpse of what can be achieved with the techniques being taught. The training is tailored to those learning, with those of us that pick it up quickly, being encouraged to help those that are not so sure. I have felt the effectiveness both in myself and in the horses that I ride (I now treat every horse before I even think about getting in the

67

saddle).

Would I recommend the course?

Do you really have to ask this? Let's take the horses that I deal with each week.

My stroppy mare is now so relaxed and happy that people who knew her before don't recognise her.

The warmblood I ride now has so much spring in his step that very transition feels just amazing!

The 'old cob' that I coach is looking like a proper dressage pony!

The little Welsh Section D is now a powerhouse! (I didn't treat this one, but her owner was on the course with me!)

The tense mare? Well, she will take a bit of work, but she is much freer than she was. She is a work in progress. Her tension was so great that she will take a number of treatments to fully relax her.

And finally, a beautiful but highly sensitive Friesian mare...

She was a challenge! She was so sensitive that she wanted to flatten me every time I tried to touch her! Tony showed us an incredible way in which we could treat our highly sensitive horse...... we had great results from this. Now, not only am I speechless, but I am also fully in awe of the great man that discovered this technique.

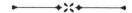

Let me (Tony Sherry) give you some background information before this next testimonial.

Tony Lee is a 30-year-old who has cerebral palsy. I first met him when he was 28. At an early age, his doctors told his parents that he would not be able to communicate and would never be able to walk and would need constant care around the clock seven days a week.

Little did the doctors know the determination of Tony and his family. With this determination and sheer persistence (some might say bloody-mindedness), Tony went to a conventional school and did well (he tried special schools but they did not work out as he thought they held him back). He also learnt from his loving and supportive family that just because he had a disability did not mean everything would be done for him.

With his cerebral palsy came major issues with the movement of his muscles. From a very early age, Tony's mum had him exercise often twice a day seven days a week and did everything she possibly could to help him. He had lots of physiotherapy and two trips to the Peto Institute which specialises in treating this type of issue. Tony has also had 27 surgical operations to correct issues in his body and to release muscles that could not be sorted with physio and exercises.

Despite all of this, Tony along with his family has become a very successful horse breeder in a business started by his beloved grandfather. Tony is known all over the country for his extensive knowledge of horses and his success with his breeding programmes.

Tony's mum contacted me following his physiotherapist's recommendation to use the EMMETT technique.

When I first met Tony, he struggled to get up out of a chair, and as he walked, the effort required was tremendous, swinging from the hips and dragging his feet while using crutches. Walking from one room to another was a huge task. As I introduced myself, I could see how worn out and depressed he felt, and he was trying to keep all of this inside himself. He explained that doing anything took a lot of thought and planning, even if it was just walking to the bathroom. When I asked him how hard the effort was, he described it as trying to wade through a treacle, and it was really getting him down. He didn't want to tell his family how much harder things were getting.

My initial assessment was that he was tired both physically and mentally. He had no muscle tone, was as stiff as a board, had no balance and was in a dark place mentally. When he sat on the edge of the examination couch, he did not have the strength to lift one foot off the floor to enable me to slip my finger underneath.

Within minutes of my starting to work, I could see that he was feeling a difference and the look on his face changed from "I think this bloke is crazy" to "What the hell just happened!" I went back a week later, and all of the changes I had made had stayed, and I could see Tony's body was changing. At each visit, the feedback from Tony was that he was feeling different, and he was no longer wading through a treacle when trying to walk. His granny and mum both told me that he was much more pleasant to be around because he was much happier and far less moody. This was music to my ears, and I knew the physical changes I was making to Tony had also improved his mental health and that of his family. We had a few more visits, and I was so pleased with what I saw unfolding before my eyes. Then COVID struck and it was months before I could return to treat Tony, but in that time his body had got stronger, which was delightful to see, and it had not deteriorated.

I see Tony regularly, and occasionally it's a month between our visits, but his muscle tone and quality do not deteriorate but improve. On my visits, I set Tony achievable goals, and he used to look at me as if I was mad, but now he just laughs and gets on with it.

He is a different man now and can walk without walking sticks. He no longer drags his feet, maintains his balance, can stop at will, stand still, bend down, pick a tissue up off of the floor, and continue walking. Everyone that has known Tony has said how much he's changed, and they are amazed at how far he has come. I know he has much more to achieve, and he is an inspiration to everyone he comes into contact with. I'm very proud of both my work and the extent of Tony's improvement.

Tony's experience of working with me

Before I tried the Emmett technique, my body was constantly in pain or sore and tender. It made life difficult, as if I was walking through a treacle or concrete all the time.

Since meeting Tony and working together using the Emmett technique, my life has changed unbelievably, and you could say I'm unrecognisable from the person I was. I even struggled to sit on the side of a bed and lift my foot off the floor so Tony could get a finger under my toes. My muscles would not work no matter how much I tried.

In the two years of working with Tony, I now walk around without pain and no longer feel the treacle or concrete. I have balance and can walk without sticks with confidence and do things I've never done before. Not only has my cerebral palsy improved, but I'm also physically more robust, and I believe that Tony and his treatments have helped me mentally to understand how to help and work on myself. To be honest, I can now accept who I am (a strong, capable, and happy man) and look forward to the future.

I would urge anyone who has cerebral palsy or any physical problem to contact Tony. You will see and feel the difference it will make to you. If it's anything like the changes that have happened to me, your life will be changed for the better in so many ways.

Tony Lee

Bonuses

What's the next step? I hear you ask.

If you are suffering from pain or movement restrictions, please contact me by phone on 07748 18745 or email tony@echtherapies.co.uk, and we can arrange a phone or video call to discuss how I can help you and discuss the particulars of your issue. I usually charge £15 for a video consultation, but if you show a copy of this book, I will slash the fee to £10. These calls usually take a while, as I love talking about this.

If you have an animal that requires some assistance, please feel free to get in touch, and you will notice a change in them that is so rewarding.

I will also give you a 20% discount on your first physical appointment when you show me your copy of this book.

Special offer

When I qualified as a therapist and was out on my own, I felt it was a lonely place; people were reluctant to talk to therapists from other modalities, and some were actively discouraged.

Over time I have learned that all animal therapists should be considered complementary as we have a lot to offer and exceptional skills.

74

We all have experienced many things and situations, which is such a valuable commodity. I will very soon be launching "The Animal Therapists Sanctuary". A place where any animal therapist can talk in a non-judgmental way and share experiences. There will be guest interviews, networking meetings, a jobs board, articles of interest (primarily if published by a group member), a forum and overall place to relax and feel part of a community and a referral network.

Having bought my book and the idea of the animal therapists sanctuary appeals to you. I can offer you the first two months of membership for free by contacting me on tony@echtherapies.co.uk